Why I Treat Traumatic Brain Injury,
(TBI), The Way I Do
Your 18th Psychiatric Consultation
William R. Yee M.D., J.D.
Copyright applied for September 29, 2020

Introduction

This is an introduction to the evaluation
and management of Traumatic Brain
Injury, (TBI) in the outpatient clinic.

The introduction includes the initial
evaluation at the time of the injury and in
the emergency room.

This provides context for the stakeholders
when they meet in the outpatient clinic
after release from the hospital.

My goal is to provide the basic concepts
and vocabulary so that the medical
student, law student, parent, coach, MBA,
patient and other stakeholders can
communicate effectively.

The reader needs to understand
Traumatic Brain Injury in the context of
the Trajectory of Life from birth to death.

The stakeholders need to understand the proliferation and organization of the brain from birth to death.

The stakeholders also need to understand the concept of physiologic reserve.

The physiologic reserve is the capacity of the brain to endure trauma from infection, radiation, heat, cold, projectiles, and blunt force without injury.

At birth there is little physiologic reserve, and it does not take much trauma to cause permanent injury or death.

Physiologic reserves increase through childhood, adolescence, and early adult life and starts to decline in middle age.

In old age natural death occurs when the physiologic reserve falls so low that the stress of routine sedentary life can overwhelm the residual physiologic reserve.

The old may simply stop breathing while asleep.

Sometime before the old simply stop breathing while they sleep their medications need to be stopped because the side effects of medications will overwhelm the physiologic reserve and cause death.

I rely on:
Beers Criteria Medication List, Potentially Inappropriate Medications for the Elderly According to the Revised Beers Criteria.

The American Geriatric Society has updated the Beers Criteria list based on evidence-based recommendations.

The updated report was published in the Journal of the American Geriatric Society.

The stakeholders need to understand the nature of the trauma that causes the Traumatic Brain Injury.

The stakeholders need to understand the initial assessment of the Traumatic Brain Injury.

The Stakeholders need to understand the trajectory of the Traumatic Brain Injury.

The Stakeholders need to understand the treatment of Traumatic Brain Injury to minimize permanent loss of function and maximize the possibility of a functional recovery.

The Proliferation and Organization of the Brain from Birth to Death

The stakeholders need to understand the proliferation and organization of the brain from birth to death.

The embryo starts with a single cell that morphs into a large ball of cells, then into an endoderm, mesoderm and ectoderm.

The endoderm morphs into the gut and internal organs.

The mesoderm morphs into the bones and muscles.
The ectoderm morphs into the skin, brain, and sensory organs.

The brain expands to about a 100 billion neurons with about 100 trillion synaptic connections among the 100 billion Neurons.

These neurons evolve under a few simple rules as a self-organizing system.

Because the evolution of the brain is governed by rules that are non-linear, it is possible to predict short term changes in the brain. However, as predictions move to the midterm and long term the predictions fail.

I rely on:
Self-organization
From Wikipedia, the free encyclopedia

The final maturational EEG change occurs at about the age of twenty-one.

I have forgotten the title and author, as this was something, I read in about 1975.

During childhood and adolescence there is a reduction in low frequency baseline EEG activity and an increase in high frequency baseline activity.

I rely on
EEG–BOLD Correlations During (Post-)
Adolescent Brain Maturation Published
as: L̈uchinger R, Michels L, Martin E,
Brandeis D, (2011) EEG-BOLD
correlations during (post-) adolescent
brain maturation. Neuroimage, 56, 1493-
1505.

It is possible to measure the fingerprint of
brain activity in adults.

In adults the brain fingerprint changes by
about thirteen percent every hundred
days.

That thirteen percent change is the effect
of learning, psychotherapy, and
medications.

The eighty seven percent that does not
change is the breathing, and other
vegetarian functions and the personality
that is stable over time.

I rely on:
Researchers Develop Way To
"Fingerprint" the Brain

New Tool Uncovers How Brain's
Structural Connections Are Individually
Unique
November 15, 2016
Contact: Shilo Rea at 412-268-6094

The Nature of Brain Trauma

The stakeholders need to understand the
nature of the trauma that causes the
Traumatic Brain Injury.

The brain is housed in a skull, covered by
muscles and skin. Every skull is different
in shape and the muscle and skin
covering is also different is shape and
density.

The result is that no two people will have
the same injury.

The injuries may be similar, but they will
always be different.

The mechanism of injury is important for
the initial treatment and for the
trajectory of the recovery.

The worst injuries and the worst trajectories for recovery are from high-speed road traffic accidents involving pedestrians, cyclists, and vehicle occupants, falls from height of greater than ten feet and injury from high-speed projectiles such as rocks, bullets and arrows fall into this category.

Initial Assessment of Traumatic Brain Injury

The stakeholders need to understand the initial assessment of the Traumatic Brain Injury.

Birth trauma is measured by the APGAR score at birth.
The Apgar score is obtained by examining the baby's:
Breathing effort 0 to 2 0 Absent weak Robust Cry
Heart rate..............0 to 2 ....< 100 >........
Muscle tone............0 to 2 Flaccid-Some-Active
Reflexes..................0 to 2 0-Grimace-cry
Skin color.............0 to 2 Blue....(+ -)..Pink

Breathing effort:
If the infant is not breathing, the respiratory score is..0
If the respirations are slow or irregular, the scores is..1
The crying infant respiratory score is 2
Heart rate is evaluated by stethoscope:
No heartbeat, the infant scores 0
Heart rate is less than 100/minute scores...1
If heart rate is greater than 100/min scores..2
Muscle tone:
Loose and floppy muscles scores...0
Some muscle tone scores...1
Active motion scores...2
Response to pinch:
No reaction, the infant scores...0
Grimacing scores...1

Grimacing + cough, sneeze, or cry, scores...2
Skin color:
Pale blue, the infant scores...0
Pink body blue limbs scores...1
Pink body and limbs scores...2

The severity of trauma after birth is measured by the Glasgow Coma Scale. The Glasgow Coma Scale and the Paediatric Glasgow Coma Scale are very important for assessing the severity of the initial injury.

The Pediatric Glasgow Coma Scale has a score range from a low of 3 to a high of 15. Pre Verbal less than two:
Children less than 2 years old (pre-verbal)
Best eye response
1. No eye opening..1
2. Eye opening to pain 2
3. Eye opening to sound..3

4. Eyes open spontaneously............,,,,,,,,,,,,,,,,,...............4

Best verbal response

5. None 1

6. Moans in response to pain 2

7. Cries in response to pain ....,,...............3

8. Irritable/cries 4

9. Coos and babbles...5

Best motor response

10. No motor response ....,.........1

11. Abnormal extension to pain 2

12. Abnormal flexion to pain 3

13. Withdrawal to pain 4

14. Withdraws to touch 5

15. Moves spontaneously and purposefully...........................…......6

Children greater than 2 years old

Best eye response

16. 1 No eye opening..1

Adult Glasgow Scale
Eye Opening
None..1
Opens to pain................................,,....2
Opens to verbal command..................3
Eye Opens Spontaneous......................4

Motor Response
None..1
Extensor rigid -decorticate... 2
Flexioon-Spastic, decerebrate............3
Withdraws from pain...........................4
Purposeful movement to pain..............5
Obeys commands for movement.........6

Verbal Response
None.................................,,,,,,...............1
Incomprehensible speech / sounds....2
Inappropriate -words 3
Confused to answers questions..........4
Oriented and converses.......................5

The initial examination will determine
whether the patient is referred to the
emergency room, have neurosurgical
consultations, CT scans, MRI's, etc.

1. The outpatient clinic should refer for Emergency Room Evaluation if
   a. irritability
   b. altered behavior,
   c. visible trauma to the head.
   d. no one able to supervise the injured person at home.
   e. continuing concern by the injured person about the diagnosis.
   f. continuing concern by the care provider about the diagnosis.
   g. Amnesia
   h. Evidence of skull fracture
   i. Bruising on the head

Children and adolescents have lower physiologic reserves than adults.

Children and adolescents are more vulnerable to complications from concussions.

Children and adolescents have a longer recovery time after concussions.

It is not appropriate for a child or adolescent athlete with concussion to return to play before a day off and professional examination and release.

I rely on:
Konigs, M., J. F. De Kieviet and J. Oosterlaan (2012). "Post-traumatic amnesia predicts intelligence impairment following traumatic brain injury: A meta-analysis." Journal of Neurology, Neurosurgery and Psychiatry 83(11): 1048-1055.

The Trajectory of Traumatic Brain Injury

The Stakeholders need to understand the trajectory of the Traumatic Brain Injury. The prognosis for decline in intellectual function and failure of a functional recovery is increased by:

1. less than an eleventh-grade formal education
2. nausea or vomiting on hospital admission
3. extracranial injuries indicate
4. severe head/bodily pain early after injury and
5. curiously, limited job independence and decision-making latitude. This may reflect a lower level of intelligence, a lower level of education, or a lower level of motivation.

I rely on:
Meta-Analysis Brain Injury
A systematic review and meta-analysis of return to work after mild Traumatic brain injury

Ben Bloom, Stephen Thomas, Jette Møller Ahrensberg , Rachel Weaver, Alex Fowler, Jon Bestwick, Tim Harris, Rupert Pearse
Affiliations expand
PMID: 30307758 DOI: 10.1080/02699052.2018.1532111
2018;32(13-14):1623-1636. doi: 10.1080/02699052.2018.1532111. Epub 2018 Oct 11.

The treatment goal is functional recovery after a Traumatic Brain Injury.

At this time, (09/28/2020), a proxy for functional recovery is expected to return to work.

The state of the art is an expected return to work after (mild TBI; Mild traumatic brain injury; concussion) is 50% after one month and 80% after six months.

That means 20% if of patients with "Mild Traumatic Brain Injury," are not likely to return to work after six months.

Most of these patients will never return to work.

The research on this subject is of low quality, but that is what the point of service doctor must rely upon.

I rely on:
A systematic review and meta-analysis of return to work after mild Traumatic brain injury
Ben Bloom 1 2, Stephen Thomas 3 4, Jette Møller Ahrensberg 5, Rachel Weaver 6, Alex Fowler 1 2, Jon Bestwick 7, Tim Harris 2 3, Rupert Pearse 1
Affiliations expand
Meta-Analysis Brain Inj 2018;32(13-14):1623-1636. doi: 10.1080/02699052.2018.1532111. Epub 2018 Oct 11.
PMID: 30307758 DOI: 10.1080/02699052.2018.1532111

I rely on:
Systematic review of return to work after mild traumatic brain injury: results of the International Collaboration on Mild Traumatic Brain Injury Prognosis
Carol Cancelliere, Vicki L Kristman, J David Cassidy, Cesar A Hincapié, Pierre Côté, Eleanor Boyle, Linda J Carroll, Britt-Marie Stålnacke, Catharina Nygren-de Boussard, Jörgen Borg
Review Arch Phys Med Rehabil 2014 Mar;95(3 Suppl):S201-9. doi: 10.1016/j.apmr.2013.10.010.
PMID: 24581906 DOI: 10.1016/j.apmr.2013.10.010

Initial Evaluation of Traumatic Brain Injury in the Outpatient Psychiatric Clinic

The Stakeholders need to understand the treatment of Traumatic Brain Injury to minimize permanent loss of function and maximize the possibility of a functional recovery.

I generally deal with the 20% of of patients with "Mild Traumatic Brain

Injury," who are not likely to return to work after six months.

Most of these patients will never return to work.

This missive is based upon my experience in the practice of psychiatry, emergency room medicine and general medicine since 1972 in general hospitals, prisons, state psychiatric hospitals, private practice and four different county mental health centers.

All the information regarding APGAR scores, Glasgow Coma Scale scores, neurological and neurosurgical consultations, CT scans, MRI's and other emergency room evaluations have been absent when I evaluate patients in outpatient clinics.

The patient does not know or understand the information and therefore cannot provide it.

The medical record is not present and not available at the time the patient arrives in the office for evaluation and treatment.

The treatment is started before the information becomes available.

The reader needs more context to understand the nature of work in outpatient psychiatric clinics.

Stakeholders in outpatient psychiatric clinics need to know many of the homeless have had Traumatic Brain Injuries, (TBI).

The rate is over 50% of homeless people suffering from traumatic brain injuries with over 20% of the homeless having moderate to severe traumatic brain injuries.

I rely on:
Traumatic brain injury in homeless and marginally housed individuals: a systematic review and meta-analysis
Jacob L Stubbs, BKin
Prof Allen E Thornton, PhD
Jessica M Sevick, BEng
Noah D Silverberg, PhD
Alasdair M Barr, PhD
Prof William G Honer, MD
et al.

Open AccessPublished:December 02, 2019DOI:https://doi.org/10.1016/S2468-2667(19)30188-4
PlumX Metrics
The Lancet: Public Health; VOLUME 5, ISSUE 1, E19-E32, JANUARY 01, 2020

Traumatic Brain Injury, (TBI), impairs memory, attention, executive functioning, communication, and balance in adults.

In pediatric populations Traumatic Brain Injury, (TBI), impairs cognitive, planning and social skills.

Unfortunately, treatment interventions for these disabilities are not effective.

The outpatient clinic should refer for Emergency Room Evaluation if recent brain trauma is an issue manifesting with irritability or altered behavior, particularly under the age of 5 years; visible trauma to the head; no one able to supervise the injured person at home; continuing concern by the injured person or their care provider about the diagnosis.

Recent childhood and adolescence concussion during sporting events should terminate participation in the sporting events until examination by a qualified health professional determines the safety of return to that sport.

I rely on:
Konigs, M., J. F. De Kieviet and J. Oosterlaan (2012). "Post-traumatic amnesia predicts intelligence impairment following traumatic brain injury: A meta-analysis." Journal of Neurology, Neurosurgery and Psychiatry 83(11): 1048-1055.

And:
There is a lack of evidence and consensus to support a recommendation for a coordinated multi-disciplinary rehabilitation approach to improve quality of life or caregiver satisfaction.

I rely on:
Traumatic Brain Injury Review A systematic review of the evidence for paediatric traumatic brain injury, and for adults with mild traumatic brain injury

Prepared for the: ACC Traumatic Brain
Injury Strategy New Zealand Prepared
by: The Review Team International
Centre for Allied Health Evidence
University of South Australia Adelaide SA
5000
RESEARCH CENTRE RESPONSIBLE
FOR THE PROJECT
International Centre for Allied Health
Evidence School of Health
Sciences City East Campus University of
South Australia Adelaide South Australia
5000 Website: www.unisa.edu.au/cahe
Centre Director Professor Karen Grimmer
Phone: (08) 8302 2769 Fax: (08) 8302 2766
Email: karen.grimmer@unisa.edu.au
Project officer Dr Julie Luker Phone: (08)
8302 2080 Fax: (08) 8302 2766 Email:
julie.luker@unisa.edu.au
Review team
Prof Karen Grimmer
Dr Julie Luker
Ms Kate Beaton
Ms Claire McEvoy
Ms LucyLynn Lizarondo
Ms Khushnum Pastakia
Ms Olivia Thorpe
Ms Kylie Wall Ms Jess Stanhope
Project administered by

Ms. Madeleine Mallee Business Services
Officer
Business Development Unit
Division of Health Sciences University of
South Australia
Phone: (08) 8302 2121
Fax: (08) 8302 1472
Email: madeleine.mallee@unisa.edu.au
Citation details:
The International Centre for Allied
Health Evidence (2013).
Traumatic Brain Injury Review:
A systematic review of the evidence for
paediatric traumatic brain injury,
and for adults with mild traumatic brain
injury.
A technical report prepared for New
Zealand's ACC Traumatic Brain Injury
Strategy.

Let us look at treatment of Traumatic
Brain Injury with psychotropic
medications in the hospital prior to
contact in the outpatient clinic.

There are no evidenced based practices
for psychotropic medications and the
medication use is based upon the patient's

clinical presentation and the physician's clinical experience.

Most patients with Traumatic Brain Injury receive psychotropic medications, and most patients receive more than one, a third of the patients are receiving six psychotropic medications (Is this because psychotropic medications don't work?).

Psychotropic medications used to treat Traumatic Brain Injury include:
Narcotic pain medications.........about 70%
Antidepressants......................about 70%
Anticonvulsants......................about 50%
Antianxiety agents ....about 35%
Psychostimulants....................about 30%
Antiparkinson agents................about 25%
Antipsychotics........................about 25%
Miscellaneous psychotropics.......about 20%
1. donepezil, acetylcholinesterase inhibitor
2. physostigmine, acetylcholinesterase inhibitor
3. Rivastigmine, acetylcholinesterase inhibitor
4. glatiramer acetate, seems to kill the immune cells that attack the coating

(myelin) around nerves in your brain and spinal cord.
5. interferon beta-1a, leads to a reduction of neuron inflammation
6. nicotine activates α4β2 receptors
7. Varenicline which blocks the ability of nicotine to activate α4β2 receptors.

I rely on:
Psychotropic Medication Use During Inpatient Rehabilitation for Traumatic Brain Injury
By Flora M. Hammond, M.D., Rehabilitation Hospital of Indiana, and Jennifer Bogner, Ph.D., Ohio State University
This article originally appeared in Volume 10, Issue 3 of THE Challenge! published in 2016.
3057 Nutley Street #805Fairfax, VA 22031-1931
P 703-761-0750F 703-761-0755
For Brain Injury Information Only 1-800-444-6443© 2020
Brain Injury Association of America.
All Rights Reserved.Web Design by Antenna

Let us take a preliminary look at Traumatic Brain Injury in Military Personnel.

When examined at one year and five years after the original blast injury military personnel manifested continuing decline after the one-year examination when compared to combat deployed military without blast injury.

Cognitive functioning was not the root cause of the persisting disabilities among military with blast injuries.

All the following symptoms were worse at five years as compared to one year after the original blast injury:
1. global disability,
2. satisfaction with life,
3. neurobehavioral symptom severity,
4. psychiatric symptom severity,

There was no difference in cognitive measures between service members with blast injuries when compared to combat deployed service members without blast injuries at the 5-year evaluation.

Eighty nine percent (89%) of veterans with TBI also had a psychiatric diagnosis.

Civilians with Traumatic Brain Injury had on fifth to one third poor outcomes on the Extended Glasgow Outcome Scale (GOS-E)

Among military personnel who suffer Traumatic Brain Injury during combat there is two thirds to nineteen out of twenty who suffer long term disability based upon the Extended Glasgow Outcome Scale (GOS-E)

The Extended Glasgow Outcome Scate includes the following questions:
Able to Say Any Word or Obey Simple Command...No = 1
....Yes = 2
Assistance Required for Some Daily Activity in Home...No = 1
....Yes = 2
Is the patient able to shop without assistance...No = 1
....Yes = 2

Is the patient able to travel locally without assistance...No = 1

....Yes = 2

Is the patient able to work at the previous capacity..No = 1

....Yes = 2

Usual socialization outside of the home...No = 1

....Yes = 2

If NO to the above socialization, then

Socialization is a bit less..1

Socialization is a great deal less.....,,,.....................2

Disruption with family and friends………………………………….......No = 1

....Yes = 2

If yes to above

Less than weekly disruption..1

Once a week or more disruption..2

Are there other injury problems that daily life...No = 1

....Yes = 2

Seizures..No

....Yes

The most important factor in the outcome
is
Head Injury...Yes-No
Other injury or illness....................... Yes-No
A combination of head injury and other
injury and illness...............................Yes-No

Score
Dead...1 Yes-No
Vegetative State/Coma....................2 Yes-No
Lower Severe Disability.................3 Yes-No
Upper Severe Disability..................4 Yes-No
Lower Moderate Disability.............5 Yes-No
Upper Moderate Disability.............6 Yes-No
Lower Good Recovery......................7 Yes-No
Upper Good Recovery.....................8 Yes-No

I Rely on:
Early Clinical Predictors of 5-Year
Outcome After Concussive Blast
Traumatic Brain Injury.
Mac Donald CL1, Barber J1, Jordan M1,
Johnson AM2, Dikmen S3, Fann JR4,
Temkin N5.
JAMA Neurol. 2017 Jul 1;74(7):821-829. doi:
10.1001/jamaneurol.2017.0143.
PMID: 28459953
PMCID: PMC5732492
DOI: 10.1001/jamaneurol.2017.0143

When the patient arrives in my office in the outpatient clinic, I obtain a complete history and advise the patient that options include:
1. Continue current medications without change.
2. Stop the medications abruptly and accept withdrawal effects
3. Increase the medications
4. Change the medications.

The context is that the patient has never been able to tell me the APGAR score at birth.

The context is that the patient has never been able to tell me what the Glasgow Coma Score was at the time of the Traumatic Brain Injury.

The context is that the patient usually does not know what medications they are taking and what the medications are for.

I have often received patients with three different lists of medications and no way of knowing which list was the current correct list.

The patient is often not able to tell me what the medical conditions are and what medications are for the medical condition.

The patient is often on a sleeping pill and never has had a sleep study with a sleep EEG to assess sleep apnea, restless leg syndrome, insomnia, narcolepsy, and other issues that need to be treated independent of a sleeping pill.

In fact, I have had patients who have had sleep EEG's and were not using their CPAP machines and were asking for sleeping pills.

Medications for pain, anxiety, sleeping pills, muscle relaxants, and antihistamines cause weight gain, tend to worsen obstructive sleep apnea as well as enhance side effects, such as even louder snoring.

Respiratory arrest and death are risks of using these medications with sleep apnea.

I rely on:
Benzodiazepines Associated With Acute
Respiratory Failure in Patients With
Obstructive Sleep Apnea
Sheng-Huei Wang, Wei-Shan Chen, Shih-
En Tang, Hung-Che Lin, Chung-Kan Peng,
Hsuan-Te Chu, and Chia-Hung Kao
Front Pharmacol. 2018; 9: 1513.
Published online 2019 Jan 7. doi:
10.3389/fphar.2018.01513
PMCID: PMC6330300
PMID: 30666205

The most common psychiatric
manifestation of Traumatic Brain Damage
is Depression.

There is little evidenced based practice in
the treatment of depression after
Traumatic Brain Damage.

The current evidence is that
psychopharmacology is not always better
than placebo.

Sertraline has the best support for
treating depression after Traumatic Brain
Damage.

I rely on:
Treatment of Depression After Traumatic
Brain Injury: A Systematic Review
Focused on Pharmacological and
Neuromodulatory Interventions
Bharat R. Narapareddy M.D.
Laren Narapareddy Ph.D., R.N.
Abigail Lin M.D.
Shreya Wigh B.S.
Julie Nanavati M.L.S., M.A.
John Dougherty III D.O., M.S.
Milap Nowrangi M.D.
Durga Roy M.D.
Psychosomatics Volume 61, Issue 5,
September–October 2020, Pages 481-497
https://doi.org/10.1016/j.psym.2020.04.012

There are investigations for Transcranial
Magnetic Stimulation and Deep Brain
Stimulation for the treatment of
Traumatic Brain Injury and the
psychiatric sequelae of Traumatic Brain
Injury.

However, no stage three investigation has
been achieved for any treatment of
Traumatic Brain Injury.

I rely on:
Chapter 17 Traumatic Brain Injury and
Potential for Neuromodulation
Shervin Rahimpour and Shivanand P
Lad.
Translational Research in Traumatic
Brain Injury.
Laskowitz D, Grant G, editors.
Boca Raton (FL): CRC Press/Taylor and
Francis Group; 2016.

Post Traumatic Stress Disorder occurs
after both civilian and military casualties
of Traumatic Brain Damage.

I rely on:
Post-Traumatic Stress Disorder after
Civilian Traumatic Brain Injury: A
Systematic Review and Meta-Analysis of
Prevalence Rates
Dominique L G Van Praag, Maryse C
Cnossen, Suzanne Polinder, Lindsay
Wilson, Andrew I R Maas
J Neurotrauma 2019 Dec 1;36(23):3220-
3232. doi: 10.1089/neu.2018.5759. Epub
2019 Aug 2.
PMID: 31238819 PMCID: PMC6857464 DOI:
10.1089/neu.2018.5759

PTSD after TBI presents in 37% of military personnel.

PTSD after TBI presents in 16% of civilians.

I rely on:
A Systematic Review and Meta-analysis on PTSD Following TBI Among Military/Veteran and Civilian Populations
Alexandra Loignon, Marie-Christine Ouellet, Geneviève Belleville
J Head Trauma Rehabil Jan/Feb 2020;35(1):E21-E35.
PMID: 31479073 DOI: 10.1097/HTR.0000000000000514

Even mild Traumatic Brain Injury involves cognitive, somatic, and emotional symptoms that may last for months and years following the initial injury.

Twenty percent of these patients will be permanently disabled.

Loss of consciousness, loss of memory, altered mental state and neurologic abnormalities after a head injury give rise to a diagnosis of Traumatic Brain Injury,

Organic Personality Disorder or Organic
Personality Disorder Explosive Type if
aggression becomes a chronic problem,
F07.89m Other personality and behavioral
disorders due to known physiological
condition.

The scientific basis for the treatment of
Traumatic Brain Injury and Post
Traumatic Stress Disorder is weak.
Symptoms include:
Headache
Dizziness
Fatigue
Noise Intolerance
Irritability
Lability
Anxiety
Depression
Concentration Problems
Memory Deficit
Intolerance of alcohol
Preoccupation with symptoms
Personality change
Apathy
Perceptual-Motor abnormalities
Social Cognition.
Anosognosia

Sleep difficulties, irritability and concentration problems of Traumatic Brain Injuries are shared with posttraumatic stress disorder (PTSD).

Exaggeration, Misattribution of Common Symptoms, Malingering, Munchausen Syndrome, Factitious Disorder may also influence the persistence and worsening of post-concussion symptoms following mild Traumatic Brain Injury.

Everyday life complaints of headache, irritability, sleep disturbance and forgetfulness may be misattributed to brain trauma.

Examination of Traumatic Brain Injury for the purpose of identifying target symptoms for treatment has resulted many checklists.

I provide a summary of these check lists for the reader to consider at leisure.

There are many checklists including but not limited to the following:

Standardized medical history and history
of the injury event includes, but is not
limited to the following:
neurological and physical examination
including
  orientation,
  speech fluency,
  memory,
  concentration,
  dyslexia,
  dizziness,
  vertigo,
  sleep,
  cranial nerves,
  motor,
  sensory and
  gait assessment.
  balance and
  vestibular testing;
  respiratory & heart rate,
  blood pressure.
  Cervical spine range of
  motion and tenderness;
  comprehensive headache
  assessment;
  neuroimaging

Standardized pre- & post-injury
anamnesis of
    depression,
    anxiety,
    stress,
    dissociation,
    behavior, and
    other mental health problems

Structured Clinical Interview-DSM,
Mini Internatonal Neuropsychiatric
Interview

Diagnostc Interview Schedule for
Children-IV,

Neuropsychiatric Ratng Schedule (NPRS),
Clinician-administered
  PTSD Scale (CAPS) A/P

Self-reported Post Concussion Symptoms
  Health and Behavior Inventory
  Neurobehavioral Symptom Inventory
  Post-concussion Symptom Inventory*
  Rivermead Post-Concussion Symptom
    Questonnaire

Neuropsychological Impairments
  Behavior Ratng Inventory of Executive
    Function
  Rey Auditory Verbal Learning Test
  California Verbal Learning Test for
    Children*
  Delis-Kaplan Executve Functon System
    - Verbal Fluency*
  Immediate Post-Concussion Assessment
    and Cognitve Testng
  Trail making test (TMT)* TRAILS-
  PRESCHOOL Cognitve Batery-NIH
    Toolbox
  Wechsler Abbreviated Scale of
    Intelligence*
Wechsler Adult Intelligence Scale*
Wechsler Intelligence Scale for Children
  -IV*/Wechsler
Preschool and Primary Scale of
  Intelligence -III
Psychological and Psychiatric Status
        Brief-Symptom-Inventory-18*
        Beck-Depression Inventory II**
        Child Behavior Checklist**
        Patent Health Questonnaire -9**
        Screen for Child Anxiety Related
Emotonal Disorders (SCARED)**
        Minnesota Multphasic
Personality Inventory (MMPI)**

Postraumatc Stress Disorder Checklist (PCL)**
Short Mood and Feelings Questonnaire (SMFQ)**
Alcohol Use Disorders Identification Test: Self-Report Version (AUDIT)
Symptom Validity
Test of memory malingering (TOMM)
Medical Symptom Validity Test
Family and Environment Family Assessment Device (FAD)
Child and Adolescent Scale of Environment (CASE) **
Family Burden of Injury Interview (FBII)

Treatment of Traumatic Brain Injury After the Initial Evaluation in the Outpatient Clinic.

Treatment is symptom oriented and, because there are little evidenced based criteria, highly variable.

Pharmacological interventions showed little difference between treatment and control groups.

In fact, studies favored the control groups except for sertraline, when started shortly after the initial traumatic brain injury.

Sertraline is effective for anxiety, depression and panic attacks and would be a good treatment for PTSD.

I rely on:
Outcome and Comparative Effectiveness Research in Traumatic Brain Injury: A methodological perspective Maryse Cnossen

Benzodiazepines were associated with no improvement in or worsening of overall severity, psychotherapy outcomes, aggression, depression, and substance use in PTSD patients and can increase PTSD after recent trauma up to five times the rates of traumatized patients treated without benzodiazepines.

I rely on:
HEALTH JULY 14, 2015
"Benzodiazepines not recommended for patients with PTSD or recent trauma."

The best evidence supports treatment of PTSD with Cognitive Behavior Therapy, Prolonged Exposure and Cognitive Processing Therapy, Eye Movement Desensitization and Reprocessing, meditation, physical exercise.

I rely on:
Posttraumatic Stress Disorder: Overview of Evidence-Based Assessment and Treatment
Cynthia L. Lancaster, Jenni B. Teeters, Daniel F. Gros, and Sudie E. Back, Frances Kay Lambkin, Academic Editor and Emma Barrett, Academic Editor
J Clin Med. 2016 Nov; 5(11): 105.
Published online 2016 Nov 22. doi: 10.3390/jcm5110105
PMCID: PMC5126802
PMID: 27879650

Pet dogs are known to help many people with PTSD

I rely on:
VA » Health Care » PTSD: National Center
for PTSD » Help » Dogs and PTSD
PTSD: National Center for PTSD

The trauma-focused psychotherapies with
the strongest evidence are:
Prolonged Exposure (PE)
Teaches you how to gain control by facing
your negative feelings. It involves talking
about your trauma with a provider and
doing some of the things you have avoided
since the trauma.
Cognitive Processing Therapy (CPT)
Teaches you to reframe negative thoughts
about the trauma. It involves talking with
your provider about your negative
thoughts and doing short writing
assignments.
Eye Movement Desensitization and
Reprocessing (EMDR)
Helps you process and make sense of your
trauma. It involves calling the trauma to
mind while paying attention to a back-
and-forth movement or sound (like a
finger waving side to side, a light, or a
tone).

I rely on:
VA» Health Care » PTSD: National Center
for PTSD » Treatment » PTSD Treatment
Basics
PTSD: National Center for PTSD

The stakeholder needs to understand the
research that supports the use of
antipsychotic medications,
antidepressant medications and mood
stabilizing medications before they are
offered to the patient.

Let us start with an analysis of the
antipsychotic medications.

The antipsychotic medications include
the original Thorazine and the class of
typical antipsychotics that include Haldol
etc.

The seminal research on the efficacy of
antipsychotic medications was the:

Clinical Antipsychotic Trials of
Intervention Effectiveness (CATIE)
funded by the NIMH in the 1950's with
reexamination in the 1990s.

Let us look more closely at the CATIE trial.
The CATIE Schizophrenia Trial involved 1493 patients with schizophrenia treated with

olanzapine (7.5 to 30 mg per day),
perphenazine (8 to 32 mg per day),
quetiapine (200 to 800 mg per day),
or risperidone (1.5 to 6.0 mg per day)
Ziprasidone (40 to 160 mg per day)
for up to 18 months

74 percent of patients discontinued their medication before 18 months
64 percent olanzapine,
75 percent perphenazine
82 percent quetiapine
74 percent risperidone
79 percent of those assigned to ziprasidone.

The majority of patients stop taking antipsychotic medications by eighteen months after starting the antipsychotic medications.

Patients discontinued medications for intolerable side effects or lack of benefit sufficient to justify the adverse effects.

I rely on:

Effectiveness of Antipsychotic Drugs in Patients with Chronic Schizophrenia for the Clinical Antipsychotic Trials of Intervention Effectiveness (CATIE) Investigators

Jeffrey A. Lieberman, M.D.,
T. Scott Stroup, M.D., M.P.H.,
Joseph P. McEvoy, M.D.,
Marvin S. Swartz, M.D.,
Robert A. Rosenheck, M.D.,
Diana O. Perkins, M.D., M.P.H.,
Richard S.E. Keefe, Ph.D.,
Sonia M. Davis, Dr.P.H.,
Clarence E. Davis, Ph.D.,
Barry D. Lebowitz, Ph.D.,
Joanne Severe, M.S.,
John K. Hsiao, M.D.
September 22, 2005
N Engl J Med 2005; 353:1209-1223
DOI: 10.1056/NEJMoa051688

Recent research suggests that the treatment of psychotic disorders has little effect on the course of the mental illness.

I rely on:
Development and Validation of a Clinically Based Risk Calculator for the Transdiagnostic Prediction of Psychosis.
Fusar-Poli P1,2,3, Rutigliano G1,4, Stahl D3,5, Davies C1, Bonoldi I1,2, Reilly T1, McGuire P6.
JAMA Psychiatry. 2017 May 1;74(5):493-500. doi: 10.1001/jamapsychiatry.2017.0284.
PMID: 28355424
PMCID: PMC5470394
DOI: 10.1001/jamapsychiatry.2017.0284
[Indexed for MEDLINE] Free PMC Article

Another way to look at the CATIE trial is to assess the number of patients needed to be treated for one patient to get better.

The CATIE trials compared antipsychotics to each other rather than to placebo.
The number for Zyprexa was seven to eleven patients treated for one to get better.

The number for Perphenazine was ten patients treated for one patient to get better.
The number for Risperidone was eight patients treated for one patient to get better.
The number for Quitiepine was eight patients treated for one patient to get better.
The number for Ziprasidone was eleven patients treated for one patient to get better.

The psychiatrist has the burden of educating the patient that antipsychotic medications are more likely not to help than to help.

I rely on:
Numbers-needed-to-treat analysis: an explanation using antipsychotic trials in schizophrenia.
Richard Hodgson, John Cookson and Mark Taylor
Adv. Psychiatr. Treat. 2011 17: 63-71
Access the most recent version at
doi:10.1192/apt.bp.108.005959

Another look at the CATIE trial revealed that there was no statistical advantage of Clozaril over Zyprexa.

The efficacy and safety of the intramuscular formulations of Ziprasidone, olanzapine, aripiprazole, haloperidol and lorazepam were compared on the issue of rapid control of agitation and violence.

After two hours 10 to 20mg of Ziprasidone IM required 3 patients to be treated for two to respond.

After two hours 10mg of Olanzapine IM required 3 patients treated for one patient to respond.

After two hours haloperidol 6.5 yo 7.5mg required 4 patients treated for one patient to respond.

After two hours 2mg of Lorazepam required 4 patients treated for one patient to respond

After two hours 9.75mg of aripiprazole required 5 patients treated for one patient to respond.

I rely on
Clinical overview Compelling or irrelevant? Using number needed to treat can help decide
Citrome L. C
Acta Psychiatr Scand 2008: 117: 412–419
All rights reserved DOI: 10.1111/j.1600-0447.2008.01194.x
ACTA PSYCHIATRICA SCANDINAVICA

Criticism of the CATIE trial was that the sample size was too small, there were too many sites with too many drugs, too many outcome measures and too many layers to the study to allow for statistically significant information to emerge.

I rely on:
Clinical Trials Design Lessons From the CATIE Study
Helena Chmura Kraemer, Ph.D. Ira D. Glick, M.D. Donald F. Klein, M.D.

Am J Psychiatry 2009; 166:1222–1228

Now let us review antipsychotic medications.

Perphenazine is as effective as olanzapine, quetiapine, risperidone, and ziprasidone.

Perphenazine is the most cost-effective medication for the treatment of psychosis.

You can expect three out of four patients to stop antipsychotic medications within eighteen months due to side effects or failure of benefit to justify the time and money to continue the treatments.

See:
"What CATIE Found: Results From the Schizophrenia Trial," Dr. Marvin S. Swartz, M.D., T. Scott Stroup, M.D., M.P.H., Dr. Joseph P. McEvoy, M.D., Dr. Sonia M. Davis, Dr.P.H., Dr. Robert A. Rosenheck, M.D., Dr. Richard S. E. Keefe, Ph.D., Dr. John K. Hsiao, M.D., and Dr. Jeffrey A. Lieberman, M.D.; Psychiatr Serv. 2008 May; 59(5): 500–506.; doi: 10.1176/ps.2008.59.5.500; PMCID:

PMC5033643; NIHMSID: NIHMS816833; PMID: 18451005

There are many criticisms of the CATIE trials. See: "CATIE & You, What happens when drugs are found to be unsafe and ineffective? Not much.," by Ben Hansen, MindFreedom Michigan, Ragged Edge Online Home

Let us look at Clozaril, the putative Gold Standard for the treatment of psychosis.

The FDA released Clozaril for the treatment of psychosis based upon a six week study.

The FDA Label for clozapine indicates that, "The mechanism of action of clozapine is unknown."

This statement is mirrored for all the antipsychotic medications because it is not known what part of the brain is malfunctioning and causing psychosis.

The FDA Label indicated that the Clozapine trial involved patients with a diagnosis of schizophrenia at multiple treatment centers.

The patients had failed to respond to at least three antipsychotic medications from at least two different chemical classes over the course of five years preceding the trial of Clozapine.

The FDA Label indicated that each of the trials must have been with dosage of antipsychotics equivalent to 1000mg of chlorpromazine for at least six weeks without a reduction of symptoms.

Prior to the Clozapine trial the patients were treated with haloperidol for six weeks at an average dose of 61mg per day.

20mg of haloperidol is equivalent to 1000mg of chlorpromazine.

Table of dosages of antipsychotics equivalents to 100mg of chlorpromazine.

First generation antipsychotic medications: equivalent to 100mg of Chlorpromazine

Chlorpromazine Thorazine 100mg

Fluphenazine Prolixin..............................2mg

Haloperidol Haldol..............................2mg

Loxapine Loxitane..............................10mg

Perphenazine Trilafon..............................8mg

Pimozide Orap..............................2mg

Prochlorperazine Compazine..............................15mg

Trifluoperazine Stelazine..............................2.5mg

Thioridazine Mellaril..............................100mg

Thiothixene Navane..............................4mg

Second generation antipsychotic medications equivalent to 100mg of chlorpromazine:
Aripiprazole
Abilify..............................7.5mg
Asenapine
Saphris............................4mg
Clozapine
Clozaril...........................100mg
Iloperidone
Fanapt............................3.5mg
Lurasidone
Latuda............................16mg
Olanzapine
Zyprexa...........................5mg
Paliperidone
Invega.....................,,,,,,........2mg
Risperidone
Risperdal.........................1mg
Ziprasidone
Geodon............................60mg

The FDA Label for clozapine indicates that the Brief Psychiatric Rating Scale, BPRS), was used to determine the benefit of clozaril.

The Brief Psychiatric Rating Scale is subjective and not objective like and X-Ray or a temperature or pulse or EKG.

That means that it can be influenced by Cognitive Dissonance.

It is very difficult to report no benefit when you are taking a medication with so many side effects and such a high risk of death that weekly blood tests are mandatory.

Look at the elements of the Brief Psychiatric Rating Scale and decide for yourself.

BPRS Brief Psychiatric Rating Scale
Each symptom is rated 1-7 and depending on the version between a total of 18-24 symptoms
  Subjective Scoring:
1, normal, not at all ill; 2, borderline mentally ill; 3, mildly ill; 4, moderately ill; 5, markedly ill; 6, severely ill; or 7, extremely ill
1 Somatic concern
2 Anxiety
3 Depression

4 Suicidality
5 Guilt
6 Hostility
7 Elated Mood
8 Grandiosity
9 Suspiciousness
10 Hallucinations
11 Unusual thought content
12 Bizarre behaviour
13 Self-neglect
14 Disorientation
15 Conceptual disorganisation
16 Blunted affect
17 Emotional withdrawal
18 Motor retardation
19 Tension
20 Uncooperativeness
21 Excitement
22 Distractibility
23 Motor hyperactivity
24 Mannerisms and posturing

The Brief Psychiatric Rating Scale is not specific to the, "Schizophrenia," of the target population. The Brief Psychiatric rating scale is broad and covers all the psychosis and mood disorders, many of the personality disorders and, many behavior disorders.

Another Subjective Scale is the PANNS. The Positive and Negative Syndrome Scale (PANSS) is a scale used for measuring symptom severity of schizophrenia.
It was published in 1987 by Stanley Kay, Lewis Opler, and Abraham Fiszbein.
PANSS Total score minimum = 30, maximum = 210
Positive scale is 7 Items, (minimum score = 7, maximum score = 49)
Delusions
Conceptual disorganization
Hallucinations
Hyperactivity
Grandiosity
Suspiciousness/persecution
Hostility

Negative scale is 7 Items, (minimum score = 7, maximum score = 49)
Blunted affect
Emotional withdrawal
Poor rapport
Passive/apathetic social withdrawal
Difficulty in abstract thinking
Lack of spontaneity and flow of conversation
Stereotyped thinking

General Psychopathology scale is 16
Items, (minimum score = 16, maximum
score = 112)
Somatic concern
Anxiety
Guilt feelings
Tension
Mannerisms and posturing
Depression
Motor retardation
Uncooperativeness
Unusual thought content
Disorientation
Poor attention
Lack of judgment and insight
Disturbance of volition
Poor impulse control
Preoccupation
Active social avoidance

The FDA Label is soft science at its
softest.

The FDA Label goes on to state that a 20%
reduction in the BPRS was accepted as a
treatment response to the Clozaril
sufficient to justify its release to the
market in the United States.

At the end of six weeks 30% of the Clozaril patients responded with at least a 20% improvement in the BPRS.

That means that 70% of the patients did not respond to the clozapine.

The patient must be educated that at the risk of death and numerous health problems he may expect a 30% possibility of a 20% improvement of symptoms. That is quite a sales pitch.

Each psychiatrist is different and has different experience and training.

I advise patients to secure a second opinion if they wish a result better than what I can offer.

Now let us consider my experience and training in the practice of psychiatry for context.

From Wikipedia, the free encyclopedia
In 1949 António Caetano de Abreu Freire Egas Moniz won the Nobel Prize in Medicine in 1949 and founded psychosurgery with the lobotomy.

Thorazine was introduced into psychiatry in 1954 for the treatment of mental illness and was quickly labeled a chemical lobotomy.

In 1956 it was known that a single dose of 100mg of chlorpromazine or 25mg three or four times a day is effective in achieving remissions of psychotic symptoms of acute intermittent porphyria.

I rely on
CHLORPROMAZINE IN THE
TREATMENT OF PORPHYRIA
James C. Melby, M.D.;   John P. Street,
M.D.;   C. J. Watson, M.D.
JAMA. 1956;162(3):174-178.
doi:10.1001/jama.1956.02970200022005
September 15, 1956

In 1997 it was known that from two to five milligrams of Haldol a day achieved 60% to 80% saturation of the D 2 receptors in the brain.

In 1997 it was known that blood levels of 0.51 ng/ml of Haldol achieve 50% D2 occupancy and blood levels of 2.0ng/ml of Haldol achieves 80% D2 Occupancy

There was a dispute as to whether 70% or 90% D2 occupancy was necessary for adequate therapeutic effect.

I rely on:
Kapur S1, Zipursky R, Roy P, Jones C, Remington G, Reed K, Houle S. Psychopharmacology (Burl). 1997 May;131(2):148-52.

In 2000 Kapur al determined that 0.02 mg/kg/sc of haloperidol achieves 50% saturation of D2 receptors.

I rely on:
Dopamine D 2 receptor blockade by haloperidol.
Kapur S1, Barsoum SC, Seeman P. Neuropsychopharmacology. 2000 Nov;23(5):595-8.

In 2000 Kapur et al. determined that although not all patients responded to Haldol:
65% D2 saturation by Haldol achieved a therapeutic response,
72% saturation by Haldol raised prolactin levels and

78% saturation by Haldol precipitated extrapyramidal side effects.

When the patients who responded to Haldol were examined it was determined that:
there was no relationship between saturation above 65% and clinical response.

That is raising saturation above 65% did not appear to yield additional benefit.

Raising D2 saturation above 65% increased prolactin levels and extrapyramidal side effects.
2.5mg a day of Haldol achieved 65% to 75% D2 occupancy.

Kapur et. al. recommended a starting dose of two or three milligrams of Haldol a day.

I rely on:
Relationship Between Dopamine D 2 Occupancy, Clinical Response, and Side Effects: A Double-Blind PET Study of First-Episode Schizophrenia Shitij Kapur, M.D., Ph.D., F.R.C.P.C., Robert Zipursky, M.D., F.R.C.P.C., Corey Jones, B.A., Gary

Remington, M.D., Ph.D., F.R.C.P.C., and
Sylvain Houle, M.D., Ph.D., F.R.C.P.C. Am
J Psychiatry 157:4, April 2000

The Clozaril Controversy

I engaged in an interesting discussion
with my colleagues regarding the use of
clozapine in a Forensic Psychiatric
Hospital with violent patients.

Because psychiatrists were assaulted and
required treatment in hospital emergency
rooms, we all had skin in that game.

One patient spit into my eye and another
patient beat me to the floor during the
two years I was there. However, there
were no serious injuries to patients and
staff at my assigned units during that two
years.

The following emails have been redacted
to conform to the HIPPA privacy laws.
The grammar and spelling include errors
because of time constraints related to
understaffing.

From: Yee, William
Sent: Wednesday, June 2016
To: Redacted
Subject: RE: TRC pre-clozapine consultation requirement being revisited?

If the inter-rater reliability was in the diagnosis of Schizophrenia with paranoid schizophrenia etc the whole concept is subject to skepticism.

The basis of psychiatric diagnosis is consensus in speculation rather than a genuine grounding in scientific fact.

The concepts of schizophrenia and mood disorders are collections of symptoms floating above a black box that we have yet to penetrate.

Mental illness is not a specific illness licke cryptococcus pneumonia, but a fever with the underlying illness yet to be discovered.

From: Redacted
Sent: Wednesday, June, 2016
To: Redacted
Cc: Redacted

Subject: RE: TRC pre-clozapine consultation requirement being revisited?

I remember when I was working at UCIMC with Dr. Redacted and Redacted on some research we were in workshops where we all would attend. Shown video of psychotic patients. then we all rated them.

It was like a competition between the various research sights. To see who could have the highest interrater consistency.

I think we need this. It also involved a nice hotel and dinner....

From: Redacted
Sent: Wednesday, June , 2016
To: Redacted
Cc: Redacted
Subject: RE: TRC pre-clozapine consultation requirement being revisited?

Surprisingly, Dr. Redacted raises an important issue. Given the complexities of clozapine treatment, it does make sense to utilize an objective rating scale before

commiting to such treatment. As many of
you are aware, a recent meta-analysis
(although met with controversy)
challenged the notion that clozapine is
the absolute gold standard in psychiatric
care. It makes sense for us to objectively
rate patients before and after starting
clozapine and discontinue treatment if
there is no objective benefit. All too often
we have seen ineffective treatments
continued because we are uncertain what
the patient was like before the treatment
was started.

From: Redacted
Sent: Wednesday, June, 2016
To: Redacted
Cc: Redacted
Subject: RE: TRC pre-clozapine
consultation requirement being revisited?

Maybe this is another separate issue but
along the line of Dr. Redacted's thinking.

We have received patient's at *** from
CDCR who were initially in the ICU from
clozapine induced eosinophilia and
peritonitis, I believe the patient also

developed some pulmonary clots as a result. NEARLY FATAL.

I remember the patient well he was admitted to Unit Redacted. In fact one of the psychiatrists at Patton did a grand rounds in which he was referenced tallking about the risks of Eosinophilia and Clozapine.

When the patient arrived here my anxiety was quite high I will admit. What am I going to do with a young man who is refractory to medications and has almost died from clozapine? Sounds like a real losing battle AND NO WIN SITUATION. Chances are so slim that anything is really going to help this patient.

RESULTS- HALDOL 5 MG - DID EXTREMELY WELL. MODEL PATIENT. THIS PATIENT OBVIOUSLY DID NOT NEED CLOZAPINE.

I REPEATEDLY HEAR FROM STAFF THAT MANY OF THE PATIENTS WE HAVE ARE NO BETTER THAN THEY WERE 5 YEARS AGO. wHEN THEY WERE ONLY ON HALDOL.

Some of our long time staff know these patients well.

We currently have no mechanism for accurately rating patients level of psychosis PRIOR TO INITIATION OF CLOZAPINE.

We have hospital policies that place the physician and nursing staff at high level of responsibility for the safe administration of clozapine. Yet repeatedly the policies are not followed. Patients are non compliant with "Showing their feces"

Patients are shoked when they come to the treatment unit and hear we want to see it. tHEY ACT AS IF THEY HAVE NEVER SHOWED THEIR FECES ON THE PREVIOUS UNIT.

Even our patients who are poor reporters are shocked that we are insisting to see.

We have no PANNS (Positive and Negative Symptoms Scores to reflect on) RESULTS OF TREATMENT

If we are to be cutting edge and using clozapine so agressively we should first have in place a mechanism to determine if the medication has been truly helpful. Otherwise the risks are not justified.

wE ALSO MAY WANT TO CONSIDER A CLOZAPINE UNIT. IT WOULD BE MUCH EASIER TO PLACE A BATHROOM MONITOR ON ONE UNIT.

I HAVE ALSO BEEN REMINDED RECENTLY THAT THIS IS A GROUP PRACTICE. WHILE THIS IS TRUE, WHO WILL BE RESPONSIBLE FOR THE POOR OUTCOME WHEN THERE IS A PATIENT DEATH FROM CONSTIPATION?

From: Redacted
Sent: Wednesday, June, 2016
To: Redacted
Cc: Redacted
Subject: RE: TRC pre-clozapine consultation requirement being revisited?

Redacted et al.

The capacity to decide who is appropriate for clozapine or not should be a core competency for all DSH psychiatrists. If there are any training issues, then training should be provided. If there is a need for feedback, then feedback should be provided.

I appreciate your question about violence and clozapine. Many of us, and our patients, also value the reduction of suffering and improved functioning that clozapine can provide. Reduction of violence is not the only reason to give clozapine. We are also here to help our patients feel better and function better.

Redacted

From: Redacted
Sent: Tuesday, June, 2016
To: Redacted
Cc: Redacted
Subject: RE: TRC pre-clozapine consultation requirement being revisited?

Sure, Dr. Redacted, it will be an agenda item for the next Dept. meeting.

I am all for efficiency and cutting through red tape whenever we can, not imposing additional procedure burden on any of our staff.

That being said, we also need to be mindful of the fact that yardstick of quality care is not how many of our patients we have managed to put on clozapine. After all, clozapine is no more a panacea than it is a harmless agent.

I don't know whether an increase use of clozapine here in the past 2 years has actually effectuated a tangible reduction of violence in the hospital. (Standards Compliance dept. should be able to furnish us with some relevant data; and I am going to ask for them just for reference purposes.)

From: Redacted
Sent: Tuesday, June, 2016
To: Redacted
Subject: TRC pre-clozapine consultation requirement being revisited?

Dear Colleagues,

In today's Department of Psychiatry meeting the TRC reported that it was considering reinstating a requirement to obtain a consultation before approving the use of clozapine. This requirement was part of the reason we only had 30 patients on clozapine 2 years ago whereas we now have 85. No rationale was given for requiring pre-clozapine consultations other than to presumably control and limit the use of clozapine by DSH-A psychiatrists. I suggest that the entire Department of Psychiatry be allowed to vote on this matter before our clozapine protocol is changed.

Sincerely,
Staff Psychiatrist
Vice Chief of Staff
Chair: Psychiatry Peer Review and Quality Improvement Committees
Redacted

From: Redacted
Sent: Wednesday, June, 2016
To: Yee, William

Subject: RE: TRC pre-clozapine consultation requirement being revisited?

This is a meta-analysis and the conclusions should be taken in that light. I do not believe this can be regarded as a "scholarly challenge" but I appreciate you knowing of this publication.

From: Yee, William (ASH)@DSH
Sent: Wednesday, June, 2016
To: Redacted

Subject: RE: TRC pre-clozapine consultation requirement being revisited?

Efficacy, Acceptability, and Tolerability of Antipsychotics in Treatment-Resistant Schizophrenia: A Network Meta-analysis

JAMA Psychiatry. 2016;73(3):199-210.

There is definitely a scholarly challenge to the concept that Clozaril is superior to other antipsychotics.

From: Redacted
Sent: Wednesday, June, 2016
To: Redacted
Cc:Redacted

Subject: RE: TRC pre-clozapine consultation requirement being revisited?

I write this somewhat hesitantly as I understand there are many opinions about the Clozapine subject and indeed ASH has a specific, and intense, protocol for dealing with this special medication. I believe the most recent data would suggest that Clozapine has roughly 3% of the antipsychotic market share in treating people with schizophrenia. The percentage of psychiatrists in the US who prescribe Clozapine (which has been available since 1989) is less than 10%. Certainly there is a lot of anxiety about prescribing this somewhat cumbersome agent which necessitates blood monitoring and a monitored system which includes the physician, pharmacy and lab. The data would suggest that roughly 30% of patients with schizophrenia indeed have treatment resistant illness. Clozapine is the only medication with FDA approved labeling to treat treatment resistant schizophrenia. The seminal paper (Study 30, published by Kane, Meltzer and Honigfeld in the Archives of General Psychiatry Sept. 1988) clearly notes the efficacy of Clozapine in a truly treatment resistant schizophrenic population. No subsequent study looking at any other antipsychotic (including Olanzapine) in an equally ill treatment resistant group, has ever found an agent with efficacy. Indeed, Clozapine is the "dirtiest drug" known to man. The weight gain and metabolic disturbances are monumental with Clozapine. However, we always weigh risks and benefits. I appreciate the fact that ASH has their Clozapine protocol. I am led to believe that sadly 2 patients at ASH died from Clozapine related GI problems. That cannot be forgotten but should not keep us from using the only FDA approved agent for treatment resistant schizophrenia. I do not know for certain, but well imagine, that ASH has far more than the 90 or so patients on this agent with treatment resistant schizophrenia. In my opinion, certain prescribing practices at ASH are not relective of those in the outside world. Clozapine can be and is started on treatment resistant patients on an outpatient basis. There is no monitoring of stools, etc. Patients do not routinely die on this agent. I have been prescribing Clozapine dating back to 1986, on a humanitarian protocol basis. I have probably been involved in the care of several hundred patients on Clozapine over the past 30 years. None of my patients died from Clozapine related complications. I have had roughly 5 patients develop agranulocytosis and all of them lived to tell the tale. I had 2 patients develop an ileus with Clozapine, one of whom went for exploratory bowel surgery and similarly lived to tell the tale. I had one patient who developed a pericarditis and survived. I have had at least a dozen patients develop a worsening of their seizure disorders yet this was well managed by the neurologist. Again, this is out of several hundred patients. The benefits of the medication have been relatively monumental, as is routinely described in the literature for decades. The sad reality is that aspirin can lead to bleeding and people have died. That does not mean we should not prescibe aspirin. Anyway, this is a very complex subject but I fear we are making too big of an issue of the whole Clozapine thing and the system may be depriving more of our patients from receiving this special medicine. If there are psychiatrists in our group who are unfamiliar with Clozapine and / or anxious about it, perhaps it would be prudent to think about training all of us so that we do not fear this medicine. I am a newbie here and vow to be a team player so whatever the protocol happens to be, I support it. I do not foresee writing any other such email in the future.

Redacted

From: Yee, William
Sent: Wednesday, June 22, 2016 12:10 PM
To: Redacted
Cc: Redacted

Subject: RE: TRC pre-clozapine consultation requirement being revisited?

Efficacy, Acceptability, and Tolerability of Antipsychotics in Treatment-Resistant Schizophrenia: A Network Meta-analysis JAMA Psychiatry. 2016;73(3):199-210.

We compared the effects of all antipsychotics in patients with treatment-resistant schizophrenia using pairwise meta-analyses and NMA. Olanzapine, clozapine, and risperidone were found to be significantly better than some other antipsychotics in various efficacy outcomes, but the results were not consistent and the effect sizes were usually small. The most surprising finding was that clozapine was not significantly more efficacious than most other drugs.

Clozapine's superiority was originally demonstrated in a pivotal study[5,6] in which it was clearly superior to chlorpromazine in treatment-resistant schizophrenia. Although some subsequent comparisons with FGAs were also statistically significant[8,9] and although the superiority to FGAs has been confirmed by meta-analyses,[9-11] the effect size of the original study by Kane et al[5,6] (−0.88) has never been replicated. Figure 5 presents the results of all single-comparison clozapine trials[5-8,53,56-70] and illustrates that, of 21 comparisons, only 2 old studies compared with chlorpromazine,[5,6,53] 1 study compared with haloperidol,[8] and 1 study compared with risperidone[56] showed a significant superiority; thus, the failure to find clozapine superior is not an artifact of NMA. The 2 old studies[5,6,53] led to a high inconsistency in the NMA, violating a key assumption of the method. We speculate that the inconsistency is in part owing to cohort effects in terms of the periods when these studies were performed because some evidence suggests that the clinical trial quality of psychopharmacologic studies changed significantly after 1990.[89,90] This finding is also evident, among others, by an increasing placebo response[93] and smaller drug-placebo differences.[94,95] Nevertheless, when all trials, irrespective of their publication date, were included, results of the NMA did not substantially differ (eAppendix 6 in the Supplement).

From: Redacted
Sent: Wednesday, June, 2016
To: Redacted
Cc: Redacted
Subject: RE: TRC pre-clozapine consultation requirement being revisited?

Given that we're an evidence-based group practice, according to a Lancet meta-analysis of 49,000 patients (2013, attached), Clozapine is BY FAR our best agent for therapeutic response in schizophrenia treatment (and violence reduction). If anyone has more credible or specific data, please forward it. As it stands, if we want the best mental health treatment for our severely ill psychotic patients, the data indicates Clozapine is our best option.

From Redacted
Sent: Wednesday, June , 2016
To: Yee, William
Subject: RE: TRC pre-clozapine consultation requirement being revisited?

Wow, that's helpful, thank you!

From: Yee, William
Sent: Monday, June , 2016
To: Redacted
Cc: Yee, William

Subject: RE: TRC pre-clozapine consultation requirement being revisited?

As the individual practitioner I reserve the right to make my decisions based upon my assessment and my clinical experience dating back to 1972.

If the matter is to be determined by a selected knowledgeable committee, then those committee members should be running the Clozaril Clinic and responsible for their decision-making process. Other members of the psychiatric staff should not be responsible for constraints put on them by the committee.

(Commentary 09/29/2020. Physicians are licensed as independent practitioners. They are not allowed to let others practice medicine with their license. Informed consent requires that the physician inform the patient and the patient consents. No Committee has the authority to consent for the patient.)

To: Dr. Yee
From: Redacted
Sent: Monday, June, 2016
To: Redacted

Subject: RE: TRC pre-clozapine consultation requirement being revisited?

This is a bigger issue than it may first appear. Quality of care, appropriate care, and medically necessary care are not issues that should be decided by the whim of a majority vote, but by careful review by a selected knowledgeable committee with appropriate training and experience, and who have the ability to interpret various contradictory studies, propose and support justifiable guidelines and restrictions (if any), and meticulously document every step of their decision-making process. Only after deliberation and discussion with the medical staff should a consensus be solicited.

From: Yee, William
Sent: Monday, June , 2016
To: Redacted
Cc: Redacted
Subject: RE: TRC pre-clozapine consultation requirement being revisited?

Efficacy, Acceptability, and Tolerability of Antipsychotics in Treatment-Resistant Schizophrenia: A Network Meta-analysis JAMA Psychiatry. 2016;73(3):199-210.

We compared the effects of all antipsychotics in patients with treatment-resistant schizophrenia using pairwise meta-analyses and NMA. Olanzapine, clozapine, and risperidone were found to be significantly better than some other antipsychotics in various efficacy outcomes, but the results were not consistent and the effect sizes were usually small. The most surprising finding was that clozapine was not significantly more efficacious than most other drugs.

Clozapine's superiority was originally demonstrated in a pivotal study[5,6] in which it was clearly superior to chlorpromazine in treatment-resistant schizophrenia. Although some subsequent comparisons with FGAs were also statistically significant[8,92]and although the superiority to FGAs has been confirmed by meta-analyses,[9- 11] the effect size of the original study by Kane et al[5,6] (−0.88) has never been replicated. Figure 5 presents the results of all single-comparison clozapine trials[5- 8,53,56- 70]and illustrates that, of 21 comparisons, only 2 old studies compared with chlorpromazine,[5,6,53] 1 study compared with haloperidol,8 and 1 study compared with risperidone56 showed a significant superiority; thus, the failure to find clozapine superior is not an artifact of NMA. The 2 old studies5,6,53 led to a high inconsistency in the NMA, violating a key assumption of the method. We speculate that the inconsistency is in part owing to cohort effects in terms of the periods when these studies were performed because some evidence suggests that the clinical trial quality of psychopharmacologic studies changed significantly after 1990.89,90 This finding is also evident, among others, by an increasing placebo response93 and smaller drug-placebo differences.94,95 Nevertheless, when all trials, irrespective of their publication date, were included, results of the NMA did not substantially differ (eAppendix 6 in the Supplement).

I will rely on the experts at JAMA to have vetted the article adequately.

I have the patience to wait for future studies to unravel the negative commentary.

I do not believe that this study will be the final study.

I am sure there will be future studies to resolve the disputes.

I will enjoy the outcome, regardless of where it goes.

Will the experts at JAMA be vindicated, or will they be humiliated?

I will not rest my reputation on either side. I am happy to be a bat on the fence, neither beast nor fowl and without my reputation on the line.

Dr. Yee :)

From: Redacted
Sent: Monday, June , 2016
To:Redacted
Cc:Redacted

Subject: RE: TRC pre-clozapine consultation requirement being revisited?

Coming late to the discussion, but I do want to make the observation that, in the event a patient does not improve in any respect when treated with clozapine, there does not appear to be any good reason to continue it. Let's not continue a treatment if it's not working, just to inflate some numbers.

Now let us consider antidepressant medications.

Depression may cause substantial change in weight either up or down.

There may be insomnia or hypersomnia.

Depression may cause pseudo-dementia with memory problems due to lack of attention and impaired concentration.

There may be agitation or fatigue.

Depression may cause feelings of worthlessness or guilt without a basis.

There may be preoccupation with death or suicidal thoughts, plans, impulses or attempts.

Let us examine the STAR*D Trial completed in 2006.

In that trial 4,041 outpatients were treated with medications and psychotherapy

Patients were treated with the selective serotonin reuptake inhibitor (SSRI) citalopram for up to 14 weeks.

The remission rate was 28-33% and the response rate was 47%.

If the patients did not respond to citalopram, there were offered other antidepressants and cognitive behavioral therapy (CBT) which had a remission rate of 30.6%.

If the patients did not respond they were offered lithium or triiodothyronine (a thyroid hormone) to their antidepressant or mirtazapine or venlafaxine.
The remission rates were 12.3% for mirtazapine and 19.8% for nortriptyline.
The remission rates 15.9% for lithium and 24.7% for triiodothyronine.

If they did not respond they were offered tranylcypromine, or a venlafaxine and mirtazapine combination with a remission rate was 13%.

The odds of beating the depression diminish with each treatment offered in this sequence.

Also, each treatment required 3 to 5 weeks to determine a treatment failure.

The adverse effects were experienced before the benefits of the treatments.

The result of the Star Trial is that about 30% of patients who are treated with psychotropic medications do not respond to treatment.

Of those that respond to treatment to medications, there is a substantial relapse rate back into depression

The Star-D report was challenged by Robert Whitaker:
The STAR*D Scandal: A New Paper Sums It All Up, Detailing the methods of

dishonest science, Posted Aug 27, 2010, Robert Whitaker

In his article Mr. Whitaker reports that only 3% of patients had a "sustained remission" and stayed in the trial, despite the assertions in the Star-D study that 40% of the patients had a "sustained remission" and stayed in the trial.

Other studies examine the failures of antidepressant as opposed to their successes.

Original Investigation June 5, 2019, "Efficacy of Esketamine Nasal Spray Plus Oral Antidepressant Treatment for Relapse Prevention in Patients With Treatment-Resistant Depression" A Randomized Clinical Trial"
Ella J. Daly, MD1; Madhukar H. Trivedi, MD2; Adam Janik, MD3; et alHonglan Li, MD, PhD1; Yun Zhang, PhD4; Xiang Li, PhD5; Rosanne Lane, MAS6; Pilar Lim, Phd6; Anna R. Duca, BSN1; David Hough, MD1; Michael E. Thase, MD7; John Zajecka, MD8; Andrew Winokur, MD, PhD9,10; Ilona Divacka, MBA, MD11; Andrea Fagiolini, MD12; Wiesław J.

Cubała, MD, PhD13; István Bitter, MD,
PhD14; Pierre Blier, MD, PhD15; Richard
C. Shelton, MD16; Patricio Molero, MD,
PhD17; Husseini Manji, MD1; Wayne C.
Drevets, MD3; Jaskaran B. Singh, MD3
JAMA Psychiatry. 2019;76(9):893-903.
doi:10.1001/jamapsychiatry.2019.1189

The authors set the stage for how
important their study is.

They state that depression is the most
serious mental illness worldwide.

The authors claim that depression
shortens life by an average of ten years.

The authors also claim that depression is,
"the leading cause of disability
worldwide."

The authors then claim a 73% stable
remission with the use of intranasal
Esketamine.

This is a major advance in the treatment
of depression.

Johnson & Johnson (JNJ), set a list price of $590 to $885 per treatment session.

Your insurance may or may not pay for Esketamine treatments.

At $590 and $885 per dose, with the usual treatment being two doses a week the cost of Spravato in the first month of treatment ranges from $4,720 to $6,785.

Good luck asking your insurance to pay for this treatment.

There is a crisis in scientific research. It is flawed and the flaws are the greatest in medical research.

Medical research is where the most money can be found. Is that a coincidence or a root cause of the "crisis"

I rely on:
Characterizing scientific failure
Putting the replication crisis in context
Stephan Guttinger Alan C Love
EMBO Rep
(2019)20:e48765https://doi.org/10.15252/em
br.201948765

In Summary:

You ask, "doctor, what is my diagnosis?"

My answer is,
"The diagnosis of mental illness is simply a collection of symptoms floating above a black box that science has yet to penetrate."

The medical literature has at least one opinion that antidepressant medications are no better than a placebo.

Please review:
"Considering the methodological limitations in the evidence base of antidepressants for depression: a reanalysis of a network meta-analysis," Klaus Munkholm, Asger Sand Paludan-Müller, and Kim Boesen; BMJ Open. 2019; 9(6): e024886; Published online 2019 Jun 27. doi: 10.1136/bmjopen-2018-024886; PMCID: PMC6597641; PMID: 31248914

Mood stabilizers and anti-epileptic medications are often prescribed for mood lability and aggression in patients with psychosis, traumatic brain injury, agitation and aggression.

There is a risk of paradoxical agitation and aggression when mood stabilizers are used by these patients.

Abilify, clobazam, clonazepam, levetiracetam, perampanel, phenobarbital, tiagabine, topiramate, vigabatrin, and zonisamide have all been implicated with reduction of impulse control and increased physical aggression.

I recommend that mood stabilizers be prescribed by neurologists treating traumatic brain injuries.

I rely on:
Epilepsy, Antiepileptic Drugs, and Aggression: An Evidence-Based Review
Martin J. Brodie,⊠ Frank Besag, Alan B. Ettinger, Marco Mula, Gabriella Gobbi, Stefano Comai, Albert P. Aldenkamp, and Bernhard J. Steinhoff
Pharmacol Rev. 2016 Jul; 68(3): 563–602.

Published online 2016 Jul. doi:
10.1124/pr.115.012021
PMCID: PMC4931873
PMID: 27255267

Thank you for your time and attention.
William R. Yee M.D., J.D
Board Certified Psychiatrist

Practicing Emergency Room Medicine,
General Medicine and Psychiatry without
interruption since 1972 in Michigan,
Indiana, Kentucky, and California.
Soon to be practicing in Texas.
At your service.

"Preexisting text," includes emails, names of symptoms, medical illnesses, medications, people, corporations, law cases, statues, text of statutes, the titles of articles, of books, the content of articles and books cited.

My copyright claim is a clam to the "original text," which is my personal experiences as described in the text above and my commentary on emails, the names of symptoms, medical illnesses, medications, people, corporations, law cases, statutes, text of statutes, the titles of articles, of books, the content of articles and books cited.